THE
JOURNEY
PRINCIPLES OF TOTAL LIFE TRANSFORMATION
40 DAY DEVOTIONAL

THE
JOURNEY
PRINCIPLES OF TOTAL LIFE TRANSFORMATION
40 DAY DEVOTIONAL

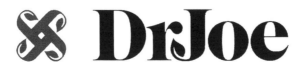

TABLE OF CONTENTS

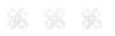 # DAY 1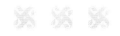

**JEREMIAH
29:11 NIV**

"'For I know the
plans I have for
you,' declares the
Lord, 'plans to
prosper you and
not to harm you,
plans to give you
hope and a
future.'"

Day one starts with you taking your FIRST step. You haven't moved very far, but you are headed in a new direction! Celebrate your desire to be something different than what you've been. Today is not about results. It is about taking the first step to create the foundation that will manifest the NEW YOU.

As you make the first step in a new direction, remember that there will be obstacles that bubble up within your mind and spirit. They are as follows:

• Fear
• Doubt
• Anxiety

These feelings ONLY have the power that you give them. None of them can derail you from your destiny unless you allow them to. When they pop up, see them, feel them, acknowledge they are there. However, realize they will die when you choose to not give them any power over your mind, body or spirit. This is a lesson you must master as you progress. "Awareness" of your feelings is only seeing them for what they are. Not allowing them to create something that is out of alignment with your desires is the key to you being successful on this journey. IT is the first step to self-mastery.

TAKE AWAY

Be comfortable with feelings of anxiety, fear and doubt. However, don't empower them at the same time.

CHALLENGE

Whatever feelings arise within your mind and spirit, write them down. Pay attention to where they come from and if they are associated with any other actions (desire to eat, deviate from your new course, etc.)

THOUGHTS, PRAYERS, & REFLECTIONS

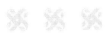 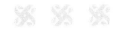

DAY 2

**JOSHUA
1:9 NIV**

"Have I not com-
manded you? Be
strong and coura-
geous. Do not be
afraid; do not be
discouraged, for
the Lord your God
will be with you
wherever you go."

Day two is the dawning of a new day. The fear of doing something "brand new" is no longer within your spirit and mind. Anything that can be done once can be done again and again. The question of "Can I do this?" is no longer your worry. Today you have an opportunity to walk with more assurance, power and certainty!

The key to manifesting the "New You" is to be certain that you create a foundation that allows your desires to reach their fullest potential. This means that good habits early in the process are of the utmost importance. It also means you must keep certain thoughts at the forefront of your mind and spirit. They are as follows:

• Remain positive
• Be consistent
• Improve daily

The above traits are necessary building blocks to your manifestation of the New You! When you practice the aforementioned separate-ly, they are effective; however, when they are combined and focused in the direction of your goals a synergistic force is created. Being habit-ual in these disciplines will catapult you to your destiny more quickly!

You are early in the process of transformation; however, in the infancy stages of change, what you do now will set you up for an amazing future.

TAKE AWAY

Remain positive. Be consistent. Improve day by day. These are the ingredients necessary for a recipe for change.

CHALLENGE:

Remaining positive in your new habits, being consistent in all that you do and dedicating yourself to improving daily are necessary parts of your growth and maturation. Is one harder for you than another? If so, write down the one that will be most difficult. Give reasons as to why it will impact you on your journey.

_____

_____

_____

_____

_____

_____

_____

_____

_____

_____

_____

_____

_____

THOUGHTS, PRAYERS, & REFLECTIONS

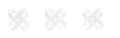
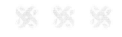

DAY 3

DEUTERONOMY 31:8 NIV

"The Lord himself goes before you and will be with you; He will never leave you nor forsake you. Do not be afraid; do not be discouraged."

Today is a special day for you. The number "3" has been significant and meaningful since the conception of human civilization. The number "3" indicates a certain level of completion that must be acknowledged and understood.

This does not mean you are finished or that your journey is over. It means you have been walking in a new direction, practicing positive thinking and choosing consistency in your actions as you've desired to improve daily for the past three days. You may not see it manifest in your physical reality yet; however, today is a day whereby change is moving forward in your life.

If you view your journey as the building of a home, you will see that for the past three days you have been participating in pouring the foundation for what you are preparing to build. When you lay the foundation of a home, the land must be levelled, the concrete must be poured, and time must be given for the concrete to set.

When the process of laying the foundation is rushed, the quality of the home will always be compromised. At this point in your process, you may not see huge results because your actions for the past three days address only the foundation—not the actual structure.

Continue laying the foundation because soon you will begin to clearly see the fruits of your labor.

TAKE AWAY

Early in any building project, the foundation must be laid. Creating rhythm, habits and consistency are what create the strong foundation that we need.

CHALLENGE

Over the past three days, what areas of your new routine have challenged you? Can you improve in your thinking, preparation or ability to self-reflect on a daily basis? Identify your areas of weakness; write down what they are and some options for dealing with them.

_____

_____

_____

THOUGHTS, PRAYERS, & REFLECTIONS

_____

_____

_____

_____

_____

_____

_____

_____

_____

_____

DAY 4

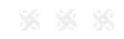

PROVERBS 3: 5-6 NIV

"Trust in the Lord with all your heart and lean not on your own understanding; ⁶in all your ways submit to him, and he will make your paths straight."

You are in a place where you've never been before! You are on your way to a new state of mind, a new destiny and a new future! This is a new scene for you because your actions and steps are calculated. The sacrifices, pain and suffering are for a reason. You are suppressing the old you, so the New You can come forth!

In order to manifest the New You, you must understand that the following things must happen:

- You must continue to move forward.
- You must not allow anything to stop you from reaching your goal.
- You must surround yourself with those who will keep you on task.

Being successful and creating a rhythm in the first week is arguably the most important thing you can do! Day four is an important day because you are more than one-half of the way through the first week of change. Therefore, today is a day that you must stay your course in order to be the person you want to be!

Change is coming because you are demonstrating it in your thoughts, actions and deeds. Keep your focus, and don't allow anything to deter you!

TAKE AWAY

You are more than one-half of the way through your first week. This is a milestone that must be celebrated. Are you moving forward, eliminating distractions and surrounding yourself with positive people to keep you on task?

CHALLENGE

Distractions are the worst enemy of those who seek change. Anybody or anything that lures your attention away from the end goal is a distraction. Write down everything that falls into this category. Being aware of what your distractions are can nullify their power to stop you from accomplishing your goals.

THOUGHTS, PRAYERS, & REFLECTIONS

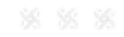

DAY 5

**PSALM
34:8 NIV**

"Taste and see that the Lord is good; blessed is the one who takes refuge in him."

If you started your process on a Monday, it means today is Friday! This could bring many emotions that if not understood can be detrimental to your mindset and results. It is common for us to view the "weekend" differently than we do "week days." The latter are attributed to work while the former is attributed to fun, celebration and in many instances "over consumption" of and indulgence in all things!

As you enter your first weekend, it's important to keep a few things in mind:

- Don't allow one "day" of the week to derail the progress you've made.
- View the weekend just as you would any other day.
- Be mindful of the places you go and the people around you.

The deeper you get into the process, the less of an impact the weekend will have on you mentally and spiritually. Prepare yourself to be successful no matter what the day is. Keep your focus on the goals you've set, and do all that you can to reach them!

TAKE AWAY

You've made it through a work week on your journey to a New You.   Are you feeling satisfaction and relief at your success so far or concern that the change in "routine" will set you back?

CHALLENGE

What emotions are you feeling? What challenges do you anticipate encountering as your routine is more relaxed? Be mindful of the activities you have planned and even more so of people you'll be with. How might you respond to them or to the old you if they tempt you to act like it's the good old days?

_____

_____

_____

_____

_____

_____

_____

_____

_____

_____

_____

_____

_____

_____

_____

THOUGHTS, PRAYERS, & REFLECTIONS

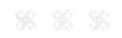

DAY 6

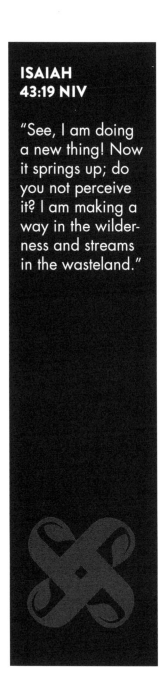

ISAIAH 43:19 NIV

"See, I am doing a new thing! Now it springs up; do you not perceive it? I am making a way in the wilderness and streams in the wasteland."

When a runner starts a race, he realizes much of the fight to win and complete the task is in his mind. He must not focus on the entire race, but instead he must take the race and break it down into small victories or goals.

Instead of running a mile, you focus on finishing the first lap. Instead of running the full marathon, you think of finishing the first five miles. Establish small wins that keep you in the race while being motivated to give your all at the same time! Today is a great day for you because you are one day shy of completing your first week and accomplishing a major goal!

It's important that you reach your first mile marker with confidence and excitement while you do the following things:

- **Run with power**—Finish your first week abiding by the objectives you set from the start.
- **Run at a good pace**—Change isn't a sprint. It's a marathon. Establish a rhythm that can be sustained.
- **Run with an end in mind**—You are running to reach your goal. Allow it to be your target.

Whatever you do, DON'T GIVE UP! You are almost there, and by tomorrow you will have completed a major milestone on your way to transformation.

TAKE AWAY

The goal at this moment isn't to focus on day 40 but to make it through day six! Each week should be a milestone that you focus on. Once it's completed, it should give you the confidence to continue and move forward!

CHALLENGE

How is your power output? Are you running with effort and putting forth initiative? Are you holding something back? Are you running at a good pace? Are you consistent each day? Are you running with a goal in mind? What is your target? What are you looking to do? Assess all three of these areas; adjust them where needed in order to maximize your potential of manifesting change and success.

_____

_____

_____

_____

_____

_____

_____

_____

_____

_____

_____

_____

_____

THOUGHTS, PRAYERS, & REFLECTIONS

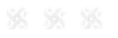 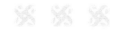

DAY 7

Congratulations, you have made it to day seven! Celebrate your mini victory, not that you are at the finish line, but that you've committed to change, and you've done it for seven days. Seven is a special number; it's the number of "completion." It's the same amount of time The Most High spent creating the world and space. Seven is the number of days in a week. You have solidified your foundation for what and who you will be.

You have a unique opportunity at this point, in the you have a 7-day "sample" of your actions, habits and proclivities. This information is priceless to you because you have the opportunity to see what you've done, so you can make the adjustments to make the next seven days even better.

Consider these three things:

- Habits
- Mindset
- Commitment to the Process

Wherever you see areas to improve, identify them in order that you may tweak your actions, refine your ability to change and manifest the New You. Allow your first seven days to be the teacher who gives you insights you have never known or understood before this point in time.

TAKE AWAY

You have completed your first milestone. You have learned and grown. Although its likely you've made some mistakes, you can learn from them to improve your results.

CHALLENGE

Assess your habits, mindset and commitment to this process. In which areas do you possess weakness? Which areas are your strengths? Write them down and be aware and mindful of your answers. Make adjustments where they are needed. This will give you a plan of action to not just complete another seven days, but to maximize your results.

THOUGHTS, PRAYERS, & REFLECTIONS

DAY 8

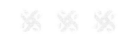

COLOSSIANS 2:7 NIV

"Rooted and built up in him, strengthened in the faith as you were taught, and overflowing with thankfulness."

Now that you have successfully started, it's time to prepare for the next stage of transformation in order that you may finish strong! From now on, each new week will revolve around a different theme. The goal of these themes is to create visuals that allow you to see where you are.

The number "8" is significant to a "new beginning." Essentially, it's time to build upon what you have started. One key to transformation is this: NEVER ALLOW YOUR SUCCESS TO BECOME YOUR FAILURE!

Don't forget that you must continue to do the things you did correctly if you want to be successful tomorrow. Before now, we have tried to eliminate what was wrong; now it's time to focus on what was done correctly.

- Consistency
- Focus
- Dedication
- Positivity
- Flexibility

These are all qualities needed for change! These are qualities you have seen in yourself this week. In order to go where you desire, these tenants must continue to be part of your daily lifestyle and personal point of focus. Let's reflect on them as we progress towards this week's theme: "Taxi and Take Off."

TAKE AWAY

All of the good things you have done must be a part of your daily lifestyle. What has been done in the past (positive things) must be duplicated in the future in order to manifest sustainable desired outcomes.

CHALLENGE

List all of the things you felt you were most effective at during the first week. Write them down and allow them to be points of visualization as you move forward. Allow them to become part of "who you are" not just "what you do."

_____

_____

_____

_____

_____

_____

THOUGHTS, PRAYERS, & REFLECTIONS

_____

_____

_____

_____

_____

_____

_____

_____

_____

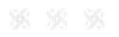 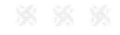

DAY 9

ISAIAH 54:2-3 NIV

"Enlarge the place of your tent, stretch your tent curtains wide, do not hold back; lengthen your cords, strengthen your stakes. For you will spread out to the right and to the left; your descendants will dispossess nations and settle in their desolate cities."

Today, we "Taxi and Take Off." This theme should generate a pictorial of the following:

• A plane leaving the gate and
• Taxiing down the runway before
• Taking off and
• Increasing its altitude before
• Levelling off

Every time a plane goes from one destination to another, it follows these steps. In your second week of transformation, allow this to be your focus. At this point you've left the gate and taxied down the runway; now you are climbing.

When a plane takes off and as it climbs, it's at its most vulnerable position. It has a high likelihood of error at this point because it's defying gravity. It is expending its greatest amount of energy to create lift and take off.

This is where you are; you will be exerting more energy now than ever. You are defying many different elements of your existence. Patterns, habits, ways of thinking and what you deem as "normal" are all being challenged and changed.

Expect the stress and strain. If you expect it and understand it's "normal" it will be easier for you to manage what it is that you feel.

Combine to climb as you move to a higher level and new dimension!

TAKE AWAY

The effort you are putting forth is at an all-time high at this stage of your transformation. Expect it. It will help you process your emotions and give you perspective for where you are and where you are headed.

CHALLENGE

List the most difficult elements of your process to this point. For every person they are different because those things that are challenging for you are clues as to who you are from a spiritual and psychological vantage point. List your issues as these will be elements of your soul that come forth during your transformation.

_____

_____

_____

_____

THOUGHTS, PRAYERS, & REFLECTIONS

_____

_____

_____

_____

_____

_____

_____

_____

DAY 10

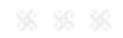

1 CORINTHIANS 13:11 NIV

"When I was a child, I talked like a child, I thought like a child, I reasoned like a child. When I became a man, I put the ways of childhood behind me."

Once the plane takes off, it begins to climb through masses of clouds. These areas of condensing water vapor are dense, and they can create turbulence.

You've taxied and taken off. Now you have a major obstacle ahead of you. In this instance, the "clouds" are initial obstacles that create "turbulence" on your flight to destination "New You." Believe it or not, all obstacles you encounter will be in your mind. You will experience:

• The desire to "cheat" or not adhere to your new lifestyle
• A wandering mind not focused on your goals
• Fleeting excitement now that the "newness" has worn off

They will create turbulence. Don't allow them to scare you because they are nothing more than illusions created by your mind. The way to overcome them is to acknowledge them, yet refuse to allow them to stop you mid-flight.

Turbulence can be rough and violent; however, planes were made to withstand the clouds! Similarly, you are made to withstand your obstacles. God made you strong and full of courage; however, it's your job to control your mind and make it think or see otherwise.

Buckle up and embrace the turbulence. It doesn't last for very long!

TAKE AWAY

This is the time of your process whereby thoughts not in alignment with your goal will be the strongest and most prevalent. It's up to you to not allow these thoughts a permanent place in your mind. When an idea remains in the mind, it's only a matter of time before it permeates the soul and spirit.

CHALLENGE

The mind is a very power machine that's central to your entire being. Success and failure all start in the mind. Now that you've been on a journey for ten days, the mind will present many ideas (similar to the ones mentioned) that aren't in alignment with your ultimate goal and destination. Write down every doubt or worry you have—anything that's not in alignment with your destination. Add to this list as new concerns come to mind.

_____

_____

_____

_____

_____

_____

_____

_____

_____

_____

_____

_____

THOUGHTS, PRAYERS, & REFLECTIONS

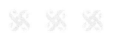
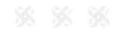

DAY 11

PHILIPPIANS 1:6 ESV

"And I am sure of this, that He who began a good work in you will bring it to comple-tion at the day of Jesus Christ."

Once the plane passes through the clouds much of the initial turbulence comes to an end. The clouds break, and the clear blue skies are able to be seen. This is a turning point in the process because once the plane passes through the clouds, that another element of travel begins.

You have come through the clouds, and much of the turbulence you have experienced is behind you. You can see your way more clearly now as you have been diligent for 11 straight days. Old thoughts and habits are slowly dying and losing their grip on you. You are experiencing a sense of control that's completely new.

While in this bright spot, it's important to remember that the plane is still "climbing." It hasn't levelled off; actually, it's quite some time before that occurs! It's still exerting a lot of energy, it's still moving upward, and the seatbelt sign is still on. Many things can happen:

• Cravings
• Desiring to participate in old habits
• Dealing with the negativity of others

You are well on your way to your New You, but you're not in the clear yet. Potential dangers can overtake you as you ascend. So, celebrate coming through the clouds and weathering the turbulence, but realize you are still CLIMBING!

TAKE AWAY

You have achieved a major milestone in your process. You've passed through the clouds, and much of the turbulence is behind you. Recognize that you are still climbing. Recognize that you still have work to do and new habits to formulate if you desire to reach and sustain your goals.

CHALLENGE

Now that you've passed through the clouds, what issues might still create "turbulence." Write them down and search yourself and your surroundings. Determine if they can be addressed. The goal is to remove those things that could potentially hamper your ascent to transformation.

THOUGHTS, PRAYERS, & REFLECTIONS

DAY 12

**JOHN
15:5 ESV**

"I am the vine;
you are the
branches. Who-
ever abides in me
and I in him, he it
is that bears much
fruit, for apart
from me you can
do nothing."

Eventually this plane is going to reach "cruising altitude." This is when the pilot and crew give the passengers certain freedoms they did not have for taxi and take off. Finally, the passengers are able to "freely" move about the cabin.

Even the pilot and crew can relax a bit. The captain will engage "auto pilot." The crew will leave their seats and prepare the "in-flight" service. Rough air and turbulence are no longer as much of a threat. The plane is able to "back off" and "cruise to its destination."

You should also find that the "intensity" levels are changing. You are able to get up and do those things more easily that you found difficult just days ago. You are able to go places and do things with a greater sense of normalcy.

It's important to understand that when a plane reaches its "cruising altitude" it has not yet reached its destination! At any given time, it could encounter "rough air" causing the pilot, crew and passengers to lose some of the freedoms smooth air can bring. Don't become complacent; remain diligent and determined. You may encounter your own "rough air." Temptations and defeatist thoughts can arise. When they do, acknowledge them, but resist them. Never forget that you are in control!

TAKE AWAY

You have now reached your "cruising altitude." The intensity of transformation at this point in time won't be as difficult as it was when you first started. Enjoy this place; however, understand that rough air can come at any time.

CHALLENGE

It's important to really be mindful and engage with the process. Are things easier now? Are you less distracted? Do you find yourself more in control of your thoughts and actions? Write down the ways you feel things are better. This is important because the longer the list, the more it indicates manifested change and encourages you. When something that was once "hard" now becomes "easier," it is an indication that your capacity has increased.

_____

_____

_____

_____

_____

_____

_____

_____

_____

_____

_____

_____

THOUGHTS, PRAYERS, & REFLECTIONS

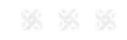

DAY 13

PHILIPPIANS 1:9-11 ESV

"And it is my prayer that your love may abound more and more, with knowledge and all discern-ment, so that you may approve what is excellent, and so be pure and blameless for the day of Christ, filled with the fruit of righ-teousness that comes through Jesus Christ, to the glory and praise of God."

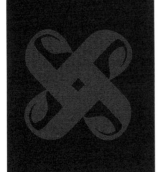

Once a plane taxis, takes off and reaches cruis-ing altitude, it's only a matter of time before it prepares for landing. Each step is necessary for any plane to reach its destination. If there are deviations or major problems with the flight plan, a "safe landing" is almost impossible.

You are one day away from another major breakthrough! There are still work for you to do and things to accomplish; however, you have successfully completed 13 days—almost two weeks of transformation! This is an incredible accomplishment, and you should rejoice.

What have you done? You have conquered el-ements of your life that were challenging ini-tially. Now, they are becoming a natural part of your daily routine. The following things have occurred:

- Formation of new habits
- Avoidance of things that are not in alignment with your goals
- Honing and refining your will (that which allows you to do the things that are difficult)

These are major skills leading you to the place you desire to be. Remain fixed on your new way of living. Build upon what you have formed, and improve in those areas where you feel weak. Anticipate tomorrow while revelling in how far you've come today!

TAKE AWAY

After almost two weeks, you have created new habits that are changing your future. 13 days of change and managing a new lifestyle are a major occasion. You have poured your foundation; now it's time to build upon it.

CHALLENGE

What actions and thoughts feel more natural today than when you started your journey? Write down all of your new habits. Each is a major stone in your foundation. How, specifically, have they made your life better? What would you like to further strengthen to ensure you reach your goals?

_____

_____

_____

_____

_____

_____

_____

_____

_____

_____

_____

_____

_____

THOUGHTS, PRAYERS, & REFLECTIONS

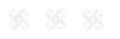 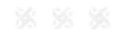

DAY 14

COLOSSIANS 1:10 ESV

". . .so as to walk in a manner worthy of the Lord, fully pleasing to Him: bearing fruit in every good work and increasing in the knowledge of God."

You have successfully completed two full weeks of transformation! You returned your seat to its upright position and prepared for descent. The flight attendants buckled in, and the pilot received clearance from air traffic control. The landing gear deployed, and your plane gently bumped against the runway as you touched down. Take a deep breath, and let it out. You've earned it. Congratulations!

As you disembark, you are entering into another dimension where you will add to the skills you have already acquired. You have made sacrifices; however, you haven't necessarily been able to see the proof to your satisfaction. You will keep making them. During this next phase, another theme will help you gain insight and clarity. Prepare for seedtime and harvest!

All living creatures—plants and animals—started as seeds. Each certain element had to be placed in a certain location at a certain time to manifest a certain product. When you understand the basic principles of seedtime and harvest, you will have greater insight as to where you are as well as what to expect as you get closer to your destiny.

As we start the next leg of this journey, view what you've done in the same way as we describe elements of seedtime and harvest.

TAKE AWAY

You are entering another phase of your transformation. You are entering a time in your transformative process where your sacrifices may not be seen as physical manifestations. Our theme of "Seedtime and Harvest" will help you understand where you are and avoid being discouraged.

CHALLENGE

You've made many sacrifices over the past two weeks. Write some of them down along with what you want to see manifested because of those sacrifices. Each "sacrifice" you write down is a "seed" that will mature into an abundant harvest.

_____

_____

_____

_____

_____

_____

_____

_____

_____

_____

_____

_____

_____

THOUGHTS, PRAYERS, & REFLECTIONS

DAY 15

2 CORINTHIANS 9:10 ESV

"He who supplies seed to the sower and bread for food will supply and multiply your seed for sowing and increase the harvest of your righteousness."

Today we begin a seedtime and harvest theme. There are several different elements to it. Each is dependent upon the others. They are as follows:

- Planting of a seed
- Germination
- Establishment of roots
- Growth
- Harvest

Before day one, you planted a seed. Perhaps you weren't aware, but you did. Your mind was focused on something you wanted or desired to accomplish. You had intention—a goal in mind.

For the past two weeks, your seed has been planted, and soon something will come forth from the ground. It's crucial that you understand what you've done. Your seed is special because it's yours. You planted it!

As you go about your day and reflect on where you are and where you desire to be, remember that this is bigger than what you see. Ultimately, it's about growing that seed. When you are tempted to give up, remember, you've planted something, and it needs your constant presence if you want it to grow. If you leave it now, it will die, and your effort, time and sacrifice will all have been in vain. Let's not leave the seed. Today let's focus, so it can grow!

TAKE AWAY

This is more than a "40 day" program. It's your desire to create a New You. In order to grow something new, you must plant something new. You've planted a seed, and each day becomes an opportunity to nurture it!

CHALLENGE

Reflect on the seed you've planted. What is it you desire? Each answer is a seed you have planted. Write down every seed. Make it clear that these 40 days are a time for you to cultivate everything you took time to plant.

_____

_____

_____

_____

_____

_____

_____

_____

_____

_____

_____

_____

_____

_____

_____

THOUGHTS, PRAYERS, & REFLECTIONS

DAY 16

**DEUTERONOMY
24:19 ESV**

"When you reap
your harvest in
your field and
forget a sheaf in
the field, you shall
not go back to
get it. It shall be
for the sojourner,
the fatherless, and
the widow, that
the LORD your
God may bless
you in all the work
of your hands."

Once a seed has been planted, it must be nourished and tended. If it's not, it will die. The people who are successful in this process aren't those who simply "follow instructions," but rather they cherish the seed they have planted.

Believe it or not, you began to change before day one. Each day the sacrifices you've made and the time you've invested are direct examples of how you have tended your seed. The more you tend it, the faster it will grow and the better chance it has to reach maturity.

See today as TLC. Everything you do either nourishes or starves the seed. You maintain its growth when you're

- Diligent
- Consistent
- Positive
- Constantly improving
- Mindful of your surroundings
- Focused on your goal

You stunt your seed's growth, when you

- Cheat
- Ignore instructions
- Complain about your circumstances
- Dwell on mistakes
- Refuse to change

Will you "feed" your seed, or will you "starve" it? Its destiny is in your hands.

TAKE AWAY

This process of transformation comes down to caring for one's seed or neglecting it. Success rests within the conscience of those who view their seeds as substantial and deserving of life! This isn't a "40-day program." This is time for you to tenderly nurture what you've planted.

CHALLENGE

Now that you understand what it means to "feed" and "starve" your seed, make a list under each title ("Feeding" or "Starving"). Write out every way you are feeding your seed; then write out every way you are starving your seed.

THOUGHTS, PRAYERS, & REFLECTIONS

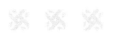
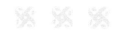

DAY 17

GALATIANS 6:9 ESV

"And let us not grow weary of doing good, for in due season we will reap, if we do not give up."

Once a seed has been planted, many days will pass with no evidence of growth. One might assume nothing has happened; therefore, nothing has changed. This is an issue for those who do not understand there are two different ways to assess development of a seed once it's been planted. One happens above the ground. The other is below.

Most times when a seed is planted, those who say, "I see no evidence of growth," are making that statement based upon what happens "above." The reality of seedtime and harvest is that when a seed is planted it grows down before it grows up! Its roots are established below before there is ever any evidence above.

This is where you are on your journey. You planted a seed many days ago, and perhaps you've not seen the evidence of total transformation. Perhaps the things you want to see have not occurred, and it appears that nothing has happened. If you feel this way, it is normal, and you should not panic. The key is this: A seed, once it has been planted, must be cultivated each and every day!

One day soon not only will you notice your seed has grown, but you will see your seed growing! Remember, once you see physical evidence of growth, just know the seed has been growing below the ground many days before that moment.

TAKE AWAY

Once a seed is planted, it grows below the ground before it grows above the ground. It takes time to see the evidence of growth. When you see evidence of growth, it's been growing below long before it's been growing above the ground.

CHALLENGE

What "results" would you have liked to see by now that you have not seen yet? List them, because each will be quantifiable evidence of your progress through this process. Once you list them, ask yourself, "Am I doing what I need to do to manifest these things in my life?" Allow your answers to lead you to making the necessary adjustments.

_____

_____

_____

_____

_____

_____

_____

_____

_____

_____

_____

_____

_____

THOUGHTS, PRAYERS, & REFLECTIONS

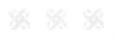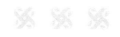

DAY 18

HOSEA 10:12 ESV

"Sow for yourselves righteousness; reap steadfast love; break up your fallow ground, for it is the time to seek the LORD, that he may come and rain righteousness upon you."

When a seed has been planted, and the seedling begins to emerge from the ground, it is the first sign that progress has been made and witnessed physically! This is a great moment for the seed planter, but it's a vulnerable time for the baby plant.

When a plant emerges from the ground, its stem is small, and its leaves are tender. It has not developed the strength and structure it needs to withstand natural elements that threaten its existence: heavy storms, frost, scavengers, insects and its other natural enemies.

You are excited. You must also be alert. You must protect your progress when it is threatened by things that could kill it and destroy the effort you've put forth. Think of these examples:

- Negative people who don't want to see you change holding you back
- Old thoughts arise causing you to regress
- Fear at not being able to fully manifest your goals preventing you from going forward

Protect your new growth, so it becomes mature and reaches its fullest potential. However, don't allow that moment to be your finish line; instead, let it to be your motivation to keep doing the things you've been doing. It won't be long before your seedling is on its way to becoming a budding tree.

TAKE AWAY

When new growth emerges from the ground, it is at a vulnerable time of its existence. Once you see change, it is new and underdeveloped. It needs time to grow and mature. The only way to get it to its fullest potential is to continue to nurture it above the ground as you did when it was growing below.

CHALLENGE

In what ways has your "new growth" been threatened. Write down everything you deem a "threat" to what you are trying to manifest. Once you write something down and acknowledge it, it loses its threatening power. Sometimes that elimination wins the mental battle of not allowing a bad thought to get in the way of sustainable positive actions.

_____

_____

_____

_____

THOUGHTS, PRAYERS, & REFLECTIONS

_____

_____

_____

_____

_____

_____

_____

_____

_____

_____

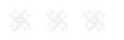 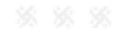

DAY 19

**JAMES
5:7 ESV**

"Be patient, therefore, brothers, until the coming of the Lord. See how the farmer waits for the precious fruit of the earth, being patient about it, until it receives the early and the late rains."

One of the most gratifying—the most rewarding—days, within the context of seedtime and harvest, is the day there is evidence of fruit! The seed has taken a long journey, and it is entering a place where it is becoming what it was made to be!

When fruit grows on a tree, the planter can admire what has been planted, watered, protected and nurtured. The fruit is a victory because the planter knows the time, energy and effort that went into that precious prize. But, it's NOT ready for harvest! It still needs time to fully ripen. Harvested prematurely, the sweetness of its flesh will never be experienced.

Now that you have completed almost three weeks of your transformative process, you should be seeing "fruit," or results:

- A different physical body
- A new way of thinking
- Improved health
- Satisfying rest
- Fewer aches and pains

Understand that you are not ready to harvest yet! The harvest is the very last stage of the process, and you still have quite a way to go. Your fruit needs to mature as it spends more time on the tree. It needs to be cared for as tenderly as it was when it was a seedling in the ground.

TAKE AWAY

When you see evidence of fruit, celebrate your progress; however, keep in perspective that your harvest has not come. There are more days ahead that require your energy and effort in order for the fruit to ripen into the juicy morsel it was made to be!

CHALLENGE

For the past three weeks you've been working on your change. By this point you should see some evidence of growing "fruit." Write down the results you have manifested to this point. What are you seeing that you didn't see three weeks ago? When you write down each example, remember there is still work for you to do. The things you write down will only stay improved if you are committed to continuing the process.

THOUGHTS, PRAYERS, & REFLECTIONS

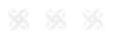 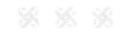

DAY 20

JOHN
4:35-36 ESV

"Do you not say, 'There are yet four months, then comes the harvest'? Look, I tell you, lift up your eyes, and see that the fields are white for harvest. Already the one who reaps is receiving wages and gathering fruit for eternal life, so that sower and reaper may rejoice together."

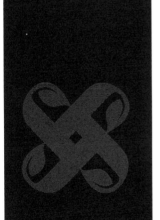

The day of "harvest" is a glorious day for every person who has ever planted any seed of any kind. It's a great day because it's the day when the seed becomes what it was made to be! The day of harvest represents hard work, sacrifice and dedication! It is the end of the agricultural cycle.

Every season has a certain purpose. In the winter everything dies, and the land rests. In the springtime, seeds are planted. The pollen of grass, trees and plants is released in abundance, and fertilization take place. Summer is the time for what has been planted to grow and establish its roots and bring forth fruit. Finally, there is the fall! This is the season when everything that has grown can be harvested and collected!

When a fruit is harvested, all of what is collected is not consumed. Some is saved for seed and replanted in order to continue the cycle. This is called "organic sustainability!"

Although you are not in your season of harvest, it's important that you are mentally and spiritually prepared for it when it comes. Your "end" is more of a continuation of what you've already done. When you get the results you want, don't stop. Grow new seeds, so your harvest next time came be of an even greater abundance!

TAKE AWAY

When harvest time comes, it's not the end of something but the beginning of a new cycle! In order to sustain results over time, year after year, you must be willing to plant new seeds when that time comes.

CHALLENGE

Prepare yourself to not "stop" once the process ends, but rather plant new seeds, so you can grow season after season, year after year. How might you be tempted to relax at the end of your 40 days? How can you challenge yourself to keep planting and sowing those seeds of abundant life that lead to your destiny?

_____

_____

_____

_____

_____

_____

_____

_____

_____

_____

_____

_____

_____

THOUGHTS, PRAYERS, & REFLECTIONS

DAY 21

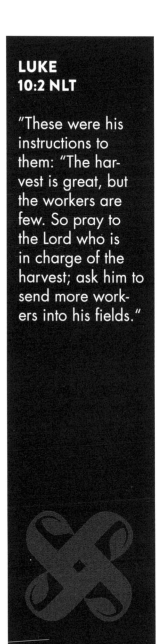

**LUKE
10:2 NLT**

"These were his instructions to them: "The harvest is great, but the workers are few. So pray to the Lord who is in charge of the harvest; ask him to send more workers into his fields."

You have completed three weeks! You should see major changes in not only how you look but how you feel. They are a by-product of the changes you've made within that are now manifesting physically.

You should feel accomplished and happy about what you've done; however, don't be satisfied or content. Those feelings can breed complacency which is the first step toward regression.

Often, when people start something new, they fail soon after they begin because they didn't know that regression is inevitable after progress of ANY kind.

Think about it: You start a project and make great progress, but then one day your results cease. You start a new, fun and exciting relationship, but it becomes troublesome and difficult. You start a diet and lose weight, but then notice the scale refuses to go in the desired direction. Sounds familiar, doesn't it?

These are natural phenomenon. Continuous progress is never permanent. We reach "plateaus," but we can effectively deal with them.

Our theme for next week is the "Anatomy of a Wave." How it comes in and goes out. Understanding the intrinsic nature of waves—their crests and troughs—will help you not lose your focus on your ultimate goal: Your New You.

TAKE AWAY

Being successful is something that will not always remain consistent. Within all things there is a rise and fall. Plateaus in life must be understood as a natural occurrence. When you expect them, you deal with them, see them for what they are, and keep doing good until you're back at the crest of the wave again.

CHALLENGE

Are you experiencing any plateaus? Have your results stalled or been diminished? If so, write them down. They are not proof of failure. Even plateaus are higher than the ground around them. Let them indicate where you are in relation to where you were. It's how you respond to them that will lead you to your ultimate goal.

THOUGHTS, PRAYERS, & REFLECTIONS

DAY 22

When you are at the beach and you pay close attention to how a wave comes toward the shore line, it can be quite intoxicating. When your eyes are on the water, the wave is non-existent. It's flat. In time, though, as it builds momentum, the wave forms from nothingness into something-ness!

For the past several weeks you have been like the wave. You started from nothing, but now, after the course of three weeks, something tremendous has been created in you. Just like the wave, you've been building in momentum each and every day. Just like the wave, your speed has increased, and your power continues to build!

This is the best time during any process: Results are being manifested, and change is evident. It can be quite an intoxicating feeling just as when you see the creation of a wave from nothing!

The stronger the wave grows and the faster it moves, the closer it gets to the point where it begins to "fall" or decrease in size and speed. This is the point you must understand. As you progress and achieve, the higher and the greater results you get, the closer you are to the "fall."

Don't fear it; expect it. Crests and troughs—ebbings and flowings—are natural. Psychologically you will be in a better position to deal with them and handle them if you're ready.

TAKE AWAY

The more momentum you build during this process, the closer you get to a fall. The "fall" isn't something "bad" but just a natural occurrence that comes after success.

CHALLENGE

What are the biggest successes you've experienced throughout this process? Have they been in your mind, body, spirit or all three? Write them down; reflect upon what it took for you to get to the point you are now. Understand that the rate you manifested change in those areas will not be the same rate the change continues from this point forward. This is a natural element of change and transformation. A "fall" always comes after a season of success.

_____

_____

_____

_____

_____

_____

_____

_____

_____

_____

_____

_____

THOUGHTS, PRAYERS, & REFLECTIONS

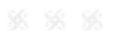 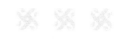

DAY 23

**PHILIPPIANS
4:6-7 NLT**

"Don't worry about anything; instead, pray about everything. Tell God what you need, and thank him for all he has done. Then you will experience God's peace, which exceeds anything we can understand. His peace will guard your hearts and minds as you live in Christ Jesus."

One of the most beautiful sounds is the crash of waves upon the shore. Everyone who has ever visited the beach can identify with this sound. The beauty of this happens at the point in time when the wave has built its momentum, reached its crest, and now comes crashing down!

This "fall" is what creates the sound. That sound indicates that three distinctive things are occurring:

• Strength is at its apex
• Upward progress has ceased
• Momentum has ended

The fall is a critical moment in the process of the wave approaching the shore. This is where you are. You've been building in momentum, progress and strength; however, it's around this time when we see a slight decrease in progress. Results aren't as dramatic as they were. Your body, itself, is adjusting to the changes. This can be a very challenging time.

Understand that the fall is an experience of every wave that has ever "crashed" upon the shore. In all progress and growth, there comes a time when the aforementioned things cease. It's a part of the universal structure. The important thing for you to understand is that when it occurs, DON'T retreat. Take it for what it is, and use it as an opportunity to make adjustments in your daily lifestyle.

TAKE AWAY

All things that have being regress whereby growth is not noticeable. Usually, we try to avoid crashes, but these are not signs that something is wrong. They're times to make adjustments where needed in order that the ultimate change you want to manifest can come to fruition.

CHALLENGE

What are you feeling in the troughs? Write your feelings down. Review each of them—process them—and explore ways you can make adjustments to your daily lifestyle in order to continue in your direction of change and transformation.

_____

_____

_____

_____

_____

_____

_____

_____

_____

_____

_____

_____

THOUGHTS, PRAYERS, & REFLECTIONS

DAY 24

DEUTERONOMY 31:6 NLT

"So be strong and courageous! Do not be afraid and do not panic before them. For the LORD your God will personally go ahead of you. He will neither fail you nor abandon you."

Once a wave crashes, or as we said "falls" upon the shore, something very interesting happens. Although it has lost strength, height and power, once it crashes the wave continues to progress deeper and deeper upon the shore. Despite its loss of momentum and power, we must understand that there is still progress!

When you lose momentum during a process of transformation, it does not mean your progress stops or ceases. This is completely normal. If you see a decrease in the amount of results, it doesn't mean you are moving in the wrong direction! You're still moving in the right direction, rising and falling, ebbing and flowing, all along the way.

Many people give up at this point in their change. They believe the slowing down or greatly diminishing of results is not worth it, and they quit. People become addicted to the strength and power of "initial change." The immediate results can be exhilarating, but they're not sustainable.

When power and momentum shift, don't give up! Keep your focus, make your adjustments and understand that progress is still being made. It may not be at the rate of what it was when you started, but if you continue to commit to your change, you will continue to make great progress! Slow and steady wins the race.

TAKE AWAY

When your momentum weakens and the rate of change slows, don't give up. It is a natural part of the process; it is a law of nature. When you're distracted by your disappointment, remain focused, and allow your momentum—what little there might be—to move you deeper onto shore.

CHALLENGE

Write down every element of distraction caused by less dramatic results or what seems like slow progress. It's important to know and understand them. Don't judge this coming week's progress by your initial progress. Instead, continue to commit to your process. Progress will be made.

_____

_____

_____

_____

_____

_____

_____

_____

_____

_____

_____

_____

_____

THOUGHTS, PRAYERS, & REFLECTIONS

DAY 25

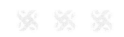

> **2 CORINTHIANS 5:17 NLT**
>
> "This means that anyone who belongs to Christ has become a new person. The old life is gone; a new life has begun!"

Once the wave crashes upon the shore and slowly comes deeper inland, it reaches a point when it stops moving forward, and it begins to recede. Once so strong and powerful, it is now impotent and weak. No longer is there progress, but instead we see a bit of regression.

Each person's experience is different. Forward progress might slow or reach a standstill; however, for some, regression—backward movement—can be very frustrating, scary and unwanted.

Receding waves are being pulled by an unseen force called gravity. The spin of the earth on its own axis subjects all living creatures to it. The force of gravity pulls the water back to where it came from.

As you become the New You, an unseen force will try to pull you back to where you came from. It might

- Make you think old thoughts
- Cause you to abandon your trajectory
- Pull you into being the person you have tried to change

Real and strong, these forces can be overcome. When you feel the pull, don't panic; however, realize that the only person who can decide whether to move forward or return back is you!

TAKE AWAY

There comes a time in the process of transformation when the "pull" of your past will be overwhelming. The power of the pull, the feel of the familiar, can make you want to give up and retreat. Expect it, but do not give into it! It is a normal part of transformation.

CHALLENGE

Have you felt the "pull" during your process? If so, how has it manifested itself? Have you experienced temptations, thoughts or the desire to give up? Write down everything you've experienced as a result of the "pull." Think about what you've written, and know that what you are experiencing is a natural part of your New You's process of change and transformation.

_____

_____

_____

_____

_____

_____

_____

_____

_____

_____

_____

_____

_____

THOUGHTS, PRAYERS, & REFLECTIONS

DAY 26

**JAMES
1:17 NLT**

"Whatever is good and perfect is a gift coming down to us from God our Father, who created all the lights in the heavens. He never changes or casts a shifting shadow."

As the water recedes, it appears that the experience has ended. If one had never seen a wave crash upon the shore before, one would assume the water was gone forever; however, those of us who've seen it repeat itself over and over again and again draw the strength to persevere. Another wave is coming!

When the water recedes, that force creates an "undertow." It is the pulling effect that counterbalances the actual crash of the wave. So as the wave crashes above the surface of the water, an opposite force is pulling below the water. The continual pull and push of energy allows the process to continue, over and over again and again.

When you experience plateaus, setbacks or regression, remember that they're all part of the process. The only part of change that is not "normal" is one that evidences only the presence of progression and absence of regression.

Rises and falls, ebbs and flows, increases and decreases, strengths and weakness are all parts of one process and one complete manifestation. As you see deviations, don't give up; just realize this is normal. Keep your focus on your goals, and make the adjustments you need to. If you don't know what adjustments to make, talk to someone also going through the process. If you do, and you're consistent, you will see that what was once weak will slowly become strong again.

TAKE AWAY

Change does not consist of only success and victories. It is full of rises and falls, ebbs and flows and forwards and backwards that create a complete cycle. Likewise, so is your change and transformation.

CHALLENGE

Break down your process up to this point into three categories: Successes, Plateaus and Failures. List your experiences under each and analyze them. What can you learn that will help you going forward? This is important because as you continue you will experience more successes, more failures and more plateaus. As you learn from where you've been, you will grow exponentially where you are going.

THOUGHTS, PRAYERS, & REFLECTIONS

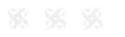 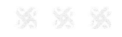

DAY 27

The wave has risen, crashed upon the shore, progressed slowly inland and now receded to where it started! The cycle has been completed! And, over and over again it will continually rise and fall as the energy travels through the wave.

The point of this stage in your process is to understand this: "Nothing lasts forever." Things are always changing. Even as you reach the points of your transformative process where you feel no enthusiasm, see no progress, and cool your heels on a plateau. When these times come, remember that it's all part of the cycle of change and transformation.

You have been working on your personal change and transformation for almost 28 days. That's almost one month. That's almost four weeks. That's almost 28 days in which your #1 objective has been to become something different and new: a New You.

Celebrate this accomplishment, because you are far beyond the point of no return. This means the work you have done has been for such a long period of time that it's in your best interest to continue! It would take you a longer period of time (at this point) to revert to who you were than to continue to march forward and reach the goal you set for yourself!

TAKE AWAY

Successes and failures are all a part of the transformative process. No person ever sees, feels, or experiences success at all times. There are natural rises and falls as you progress. This is important to understand now because as you continue to cycle through, you will understand it for what it is. Those points of regress or stagnation are small in the large scope of your destiny.

CHALLENGE

What has been your greatest celebration or your most challenging element of this process thus far? What have you had to work the hardest to overcome and defeat? And, how have you celebrated your success. Write them down and rest secure that the cycle will continue. Remember that Jesus is the same yesterday, today, and forever.

THOUGHTS, PRAYERS, & REFLECTIONS

DAY 28

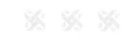

JEREMIAH 29:11 NLT

"For I know the plans I have for you," says the LORD. "They are plans for good and not for disaster, to give you a future and a hope."

One month of diligence is now behind you. You have manifested results: physical, emotional and spiritual. The end is in sight.

At this point you have experienced every element of transformation:

- Success
- Progress
- Stagnation (Plateaus)
- Failures

From this point forward, your process of transformation will be a constant recycling of the aforementioned things. You are in a good place because you have experienced all of them; therefore, when they arise again, you will neither be caught unaware, nor will you allow them to control you or your thoughts.

You have learned so much about yourself in the last 28 days that you have, in essence, gone from a child to an adult. Your insight is greater, and during the next seven days, you'll use it to enhance your consistency, focus, positivity and ability to learn from any mistakes you feel like you've made in the last 27 days.

If you allow the aforementioned items to be your points of focus, you will maximize the results you've experienced so far.

TAKE AWAY

At this point, you have built upon your firm foundation. You have seen every element of transformation. Now it's time to continue to add to what you know in order to refine your process and enhance your results.

CHALLENGE

If you had to restart this process, what would you do differently? Write it down. Use the remaining 11 days as an opportunity to do those things in a better way.

_____

_____

_____

_____

_____

_____

_____

_____

_____

_____

_____

_____

_____

_____

THOUGHTS, PRAYERS, & REFLECTIONS

DAY 29

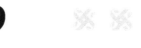

**JOSHUA
1:9 NLT**

"This is my com-
mand—be strong
and courageous!
Do not be afraid
or discouraged.
For the LORD your
God is with you
wherever you go."

Every man and woman starts life as a baby. There is no other way to experience humanity. When we come into the world, we are helpless and completely dependent upon someone else's care. A baby's livelihood requires that someone else provide for his or her many needs:

- To be fed
- To be cleaned
- To be protected
- To be taught
- To be guided
- To be corrected

If you reflect upon your own life, you were given a parent or guardian who provided these for you. Without that person, you wouldn't be where you are today!

Likewise, when a person starts a process of transformation, they are in essence being born again. It's difficult to change and transform without provision and guidance. When you first began the process, you were given and taught everything that you needed. You were helpless, confused and unsure as to what to do. For this reason, the initial part of the process was difficult.

You experienced challenges. Failure in the transformative process comes because many people attempt to change by themselves. We have made it this far together. I want to congratulate you for making it past your "rebirth!" Now, it's on to the next stage as you take your final steps toward your destiny.

TAKE AWAY

Every person goes through a "rebirth" when proceeding through any process of transformation. The nature of rebirth causes the person to be vulnerable and helpless which is why it's important to not attempt any process of transformation without help or guidance.

CHALLENGE

What do you know now that you did not know when you started four weeks ago? Think about this, and write down some things you have learned about yourself, life and this process of transformation.

_____

_____

_____

_____

_____

_____

_____

_____

_____

_____

_____

_____

_____

THOUGHTS, PRAYERS, & REFLECTIONS

DAY 30

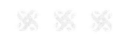

PHILIPPIANS 4:13 KJV

"I can do all things through Christ which strengtheneth me."

Once a child is born and has some time to grow, he changes from being a "new born" to a toddler. The child begins to move and understand more about himself and what he wants and needs. He still is dependent upon someone else to care for his basic needs.

You are now a toddler. You are no longer "new" to the process of change, but you are far from being an adult or completely independent. It's important that you understand this because in 10 more days—once you reach day 40—it may feel like you have "arrived." In truth, you will have only scratched the surface.

Many times "change" lasts for a short period of time—regardless of the area changed. People relapse, and all the weight returns or the old way of thinking comes back. This occurs because they are still at the toddler stage, but they live their lives as though they are adults. They put themselves around people and situations they are not ready to be exposed to.

It's important that you celebrate your change but also keep it in perspective. Although you are growing up in your process, you have not become an adult! Let's understand where we are so that we may keep focused on a full transformation and not a partial one.

TAKE AWAY

When infants become toddlers, they may have more mobility, but they still need guidance and protection from themselves and their surroundings. It's important that you realize this is where you are. Celebrate your transformation but realize there is room for you to grow.

CHALLENGE

What issues are you experiencing in your process? What things have you been working on that are still obstacles or problems for you? Write them down. This is important because they will show you those things you need to focus on to transcend to the next level of development in your transformative process.

_____

_____

_____

_____

_____

_____

_____

_____

_____

_____

_____

_____

THOUGHTS, PRAYERS, & REFLECTIONS

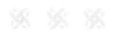 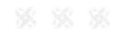

DAY 31

**ISAIAH
41:10 KJV**

"Fear thou not;
for I am with thee:
be not dismayed;
for I am thy God:
I will strengthen
thee; yea, I will
help thee; yea, I
will uphold thee
with the right hand
of my righteous-
ness."

Once a child passes the toddler stage, the next stage whereby change comes is adolescence. This is, in essence, the final stage before adulthood. When a child reaches adolescence, for the first time the concept of "independence" is a reality. Individuals are able to do many things they could not do in any other stage of life:

- Defend themselves
- Feed themselves
- Think for themselves
- Provide for themselves

This person is "able" to do most of what an adult can; however, the person is still not an adult! Adolescence, because of this new independence, leads many people astray!

Once you complete your 40-day process, you will have reached adolescence. You will understand yourself and your future like never before. You will be able to move forward because you have now prepared yourself for future issues or obstacles that may arise.

The issue is you haven't been at this stage for a long time, and you have not achieved the highest form of the human experience (adulthood). This means that when you finish the process, although you are able to navigate life in a desirable way, there is still room to grow and progress.

TAKE AWAY

By the time you finish his process, you will (metaphorically speaking) be an "adult-escent." You will be to the point where you have independence; however, there is still room to grow and progress. It's important for you to understand this now, so when you complete the process you understand there is still work for you to accomplish!

CHALLENGE

When you complete this process, what other ways can you grow and progress? There are things you can do "better" that can be points of focus once you finish. What are they? What are the areas you can improve in now? List them, so you create targets once the process ends.

_____

_____

_____

_____

_____

_____

_____

_____

_____

_____

THOUGHTS, PRAYERS, & REFLECTIONS

DAY 32

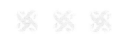

2 TIMOTHY 1:7 KJV

"For God hath not given us the spirit of fear; but of power, and of love, and of a sound mind."

All children long for the day when they become "grown-ups." Children see the advantages of being an adult that are not available to them, and they are motivated to become adults to gain those advantages:

- Freedom
- Ability to go and come as they desire
- Solitude
- Freedom to be who they desire to be

Although adulthood has its challenges, it should be your goal once you complete this process. Desire to be able to regulate yourself: control your actions, thoughts, and desires.

When I started the process, I weighed 330 lbs. and was completely addicted to food. When I first started to lose weight, many things tempted me:

- The smell of food
- Food commercials
- The sight of pastries
- The smell of bread baking

I knew I needed to avoid them. I struggled because I was only an infant in the process. However, I grew and reached adulthood where I developed power over these temptations. This should be your goal as you get closer to the manifestation of your destiny: your New You!

TAKE AWAY

Every child desires to become an adult. In adulthood, people have freedoms they are unable to possess when they are children. This is where you should desire to be one day. The only way to get to this point of your process is to stay committed to change even once the 40 days have "ended."

CHALLENGE

List the items in your life now that lead you away from the lifestyle you desire to have. In today's devotion, you saw the things that caused me issues. What are the things that bring you issues? Write them down. Allow these things to be the items you work on. Also, as you grow, notice when they stop having power over you. When this happens, it will be a sign you are becoming an adult.

_____

_____

_____

_____

_____

_____

_____

_____

_____

_____

_____

_____

THOUGHTS, PRAYERS, & REFLECTIONS

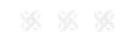

DAY 33

EPHESIANS 6:10 KJV

"Finally, my brethren, be strong in the Lord, and in the power of his might."

Adulthood is not without its challenges and difficulties. As a matter of fact, it's quite the opposite. With freedom and independence comes great responsibility. The difference between being a child and an adult is that the adult has gained knowledge, power and understanding to better handle life's challenges and difficulties.

In time, you will reach "adulthood" as it relates to your transformative process. You will be able to navigate issues, obstacles and setbacks better than you ever have. It's important for you to understand that at this point in your transformation you are building this capacity. It may not make sense to you, but in time it will!

When you were a child, you were taught certain things: how to say "please" and "thank you," and clean your room, what to eat and what types of people to avoid. You embraced values and morals that created the fiber of the person you have now become. Your ability to do those things as a child is what makes you the adult that you are now. Does that make sense?

Realizing the type of "child" you are now will impact the "adult" you become. Your ability to be diligent, focused, steadfast and unwavering will lead you to be who you desire to be. There will be many obstacles that come with adulthood; however, right now, you are working on the capacity to become the person you need to be in order to address them when they do!

TAKE AWAY

What you learn as a child will impact the adult you become. It's important that you take where you are right now seriously. Although you are only 33 days into your process, you are creating the skin, bones, and moral fiber of the person you will become.

CHALLENGE

What do you see yourself becoming one year from today? How do you want your life to be or look different? Write down each goal you have and the things you want for yourself mentally, physically and spiritually. Than ask yourself, "What can I do now in order to manifest those things in my life?" This challenge will help you focus on today in order maximize your tomorrow.

THOUGHTS, PRAYERS, & REFLECTIONS

DAY 34

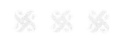

**PSALM
37:24 KJV**

"Though he fall,
he shall not be
utterly cast down:
for the LORD
upholdeth him
with his hand."

When a person becomes an adult, the next stage of life is to become a "wise" adult. Many people use "wise" and "old" interchangeably and assume that the older we become the wiser we become. This is not always the case. There are many people who are "old" but lack wisdom. Wisdom results in adjusting one's perspective and understanding because of experience.

One day, it should be your desire to become a "wise" man or woman. All of your mistakes, trials, tribulations, setbacks, victories, defeats, wins and losses have led you to a place where you otherwise would not be without them. A wise man is one who can grow from "good" and "bad" things. The wise man understands "good" and "bad" are relative to how each person defines them.

When wisdom is gained, it should not be hoarded; it should be shared. Whatever you're learning from your process, use it to help others who are as you were. Share it with family members, friends and even strangers. Mentor those who are young and learning; it will lead to the positive evolution of the masses.

Within the process we have created for you, there will be many opportunities to influence future groups who traverse the same road you are on now. We hope you make the decision to lead—if not with us, within the confines of the space and season you are in right now.

TAKE AWAY

"Wisdom" is knowledge gained through experience. When you complete this process and continue on to "adulthood" you should one day desire to reach a stage of "wisdom." This means you'll have been able to apply what you have learned to manifest the life you want.

CHALLENGE

What could you teach someone right now based upon what you've learned about yourself over the past 34 days? Write down each lesson and who you could share it with.

_____

_____

_____

_____

_____

_____

_____

_____

_____

_____

_____

_____

_____

THOUGHTS, PRAYERS, & REFLECTIONS

DAY 35

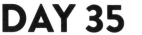

**ISAIAH
40:29-31 KJV**

"He giveth power to the faint; and to them that have no might he increaseth strength. ³⁰Even the youths shall faint and be weary, and the young men shall utterly fall: ³¹But they that wait upon the LORD shall renew their strength; they shall mount up with wings as eagles; they shall run, and not be weary; and they shall walk, and not faint."

Today is a special day for you! You have successfully completed five weeks of change! Think about that. You are five weeks closer to being who you want to be: the New You. Celebrate what you have done but anticipate many great things that are ahead!

Within the context of this process, five weeks of transformation have manifested many noticeable changes. At this point, you can clearly see many benefits:

• Noticeable weight loss
• Fewer aches and pains
• More restorative sleep
• A more positive outlook on life
• Feeling closer to God

Even if you've made mistakes or had brief setbacks, the benefits make it worth it. If they are, it is a good indication that your transformation is rock-solid.

When you look at your results, be happy you were able to manifest them as you did. Realize, though, that there is no guarantee you will keep them. This can be a troubling thought. But it's a good thought because the reality is that these changes can leave if you are not willing to do what needs to be done to keep them and build upon what you have been able to accomplish! Keep pressing forward!

TAKE AWAY

At this point of your process, you should be reaping many benefits due to the changes you've made in your life. The changes should be physical, spiritual, emotional and mental. Allow these changes to motivate you to keep moving forward.

CHALLENGE

Out of all of the benefits that we covered in day 35, which have you benefited from the least? Once you answer the question, ask yourself, "What can I do now to make adjustment to manifest the change I want to see?" Although you are five days away from the "end" of your process, you can allow your answer to be a goal you deliberately set.

THOUGHTS, PRAYERS, & REFLECTIONS

DAY 36

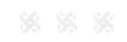

ISAIAH 41:10 KJV

"Fear thou not; for I am with thee: be not dismayed; for I am thy God: I will strengthen thee; yea, I will help thee; yea, I will uphold thee with the right hand of my righteousness."

When a mother eagle has hatched her eaglets, they remain in the nest until it's time to fly. They don't know when that time is, but the mother does! She prepared the nest for this time before they were even born. She used branches and stern wooden limbs as the "base." She then filled the nest with feathers and other materials to make it comfortable.

As the eaglets grow, they move around and dislodge the soft feathers, and the young eagles are exposed to the stern, hard limbs at the base of the nest. This design makes the young eagles uncomfortable which encourages them to leave the nest by learning how to fly!

You are days away from "leaving your nest." You've been in the comfort of a group, with a coach, inspired on a daily basis. Soon those safeguards will not be present. You will be on your own; you must learn how to fly! This can make entering the last stretch of the process troubling. You may wonder if you can be successful on your own. You might even be afraid.

Fear of the unknown strikes at the core of any human being. It's uncomfortable. But comfort does not manifest growth! That happens by exploring those places you've never been and doing what you've never done. How much have you learned, and how much have you really changed? This question can only be answered once you exit the nest and learn how to fly!

TAKE AWAY

Growth cannot occur in a season of total comfort. Only when we are stretched and squeezed, poked and prodded, are we able to grow and become who we desire to be. When this process "ends," you will have a great opportunity to experience what you otherwise would have avoided.

CHALLENGE

What are your biggest fears once you're on your own? Do you believe there are things you will not be able to do or accomplish? Write them down. Create a list of things you can use as points of focus for your continual growth and improvement.

_____

_____

_____   **THOUGHTS,
                                         PRAYERS, &
_____   REFLECTIONS**

_____

_____

_____

_____

_____

_____

_____

_____

_____

DAY 37

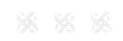

When the day comes for the eaglets to learn how to fly, the mother eagle picks them up in her large talons. She takes them far away from the nest, high into the sky to prepare them for their first lesson. Gripped securely in their mother's talons, they are unaware as to where they are going.

Once the mother eagle gets to the height she desires, without warning, she eases her grip! It's in the release and the fall that they are really able to learn how to fly!

Now fledglings, they are forced to endure a feeling they have never felt before. The sensation of falling is real to them at this moment. The young eagles plummet through the air, flapping their wings erratically and in an uncoordinated way.

We learn lessons more efficiently when we are forced to learn them! Many would never be learned if life didn't place us in uncomfortable positions. These moments can be crucial if one possesses the right mindset.

You may feel that you are "falling." If you feel like this, post day 40, its OK, completely normal! It's all part of your process. It's in the feeling of "falling" you will learn how to fly. When your time to fly comes, don't worry! Just fly!

TAKE AWAY

When this process "ends" you may feel like you are falling; however, know that it will provide a great experience to learn and improve upon yourself!

CHALLENGE

Think of three lessons you've learned in life whereby your situation or circumstance forced you to learn something you otherwise would not. This could be the loss of a loved one or a divorce; perhaps even a failed business. List your experiences, and reflect upon the lesson you learned in each one.

THOUGHTS, PRAYERS, & REFLECTIONS

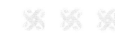

DAY 38

PHILIPPIANS 1:9-11 KJV

"And this I pray, that your love may abound yet more and more in knowledge and in all judgment; ¹⁰That ye may approve things that are excellent; that ye may be sincere and without offence till the day of Christ; ¹¹Being filled with the fruits of righteousness, which are by Jesus Christ, unto the glory and praise of God."

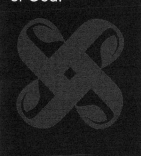

As the fledgling helplessly flaps its wings, the action is foreign and unconscious. Before long, something happens, and its movements become more coordinated. The aimless flapping turns to flying. Perhaps the learning process takes many times of falling, but in time the young eagle learns!

Anyone observing may wonder how the young eagle knows to do this. What makes the young eagle fly in a coordinated way? The answer is instinct! All along, there was something inside the young eagle that lead him to be successful in his efforts.

When you finish your process, instinct will kick in! You have been taught much. Because this is day 38, you have experienced and received many lessons that are engrained within your consciousness:

• Be positive
• Be consistent
• Surround yourself with positive people
• Embrace discomfort
• Learn from your mistakes

When you find yourself in a difficult place in your quest to be your best, these lessons will come to the forefront of your mind. If you hold onto them as you have up to now, they will meet you when you need them the most!

TAKE AWAY

There are many things you've been taught over the past 38 days. The lessons you have learned have impacted you in ways you may be unaware of now. In time, you will reflect on lessons you've learned, and you will be able to recall them when you need them most.

CHALLENGE

What lessons have had the biggest impact on you at this point? Write them down. Seek to understand not only what they are but why they've impacted your life as they have.

THOUGHTS, PRAYERS, & REFLECTIONS

DAY 39

**PSALM
121:7–8 KJV**

"The LORD shall preserve thee from all evil: he shall preserve thy soul. 8The LORD shall preserve thy going out and thy coming in from this time forth, and even for evermore."

I have been leading transformative groups for the past eight years. This has been a field of ministry whereby I have witnessed the transformations of many people. One of the most asked questions from participants is this: "What am I going to do when this process is over?" Many people fear that the temptations of their old selves will overtake the people they have become. If you share this fear, allow me to tell you one last story about the mother eagle and her young.

When Mother Eagle drops her young, they fall through the air trying their best to learn how to fly. Some learn, and others fall. The entire time, though, Mother Eagle is watching from above!

Instinctively, she cares for her young, and she is watching every moment. She remains out of sight, but if necessary, and just in the nick of time, she will swoop down to capture them.

The Almighty God, who has created you, me and all things will continue to watch over you. While those fledglings are falling, they never see their mother, but she is there! You might not see God or feel His presence at times, but He will be there every step of the way!

Allow this fact to ease your angst. Know that God is with you watching over you from above. You will be just fine, and when you need Him, He will be right there!

TAKE AWAY

At this moment, it is normal for a person to feel angst about the things that could go wrong. This is to be expected; however, we must remember, God is watching over us. No matter what happens, God will be there!

CHALLENGE

Think back on a time in your life when God showed up for you when you needed him the most. Reflect on it. This is important because God will show Himself to you again at a time when you most need Him. This exercise reiterates God's love for you.

THOUGHTS, PRAYERS, & REFLECTIONS

DAY 40

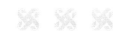

You've made it 40 days! You have done something most are not able to do, and that is change! Your road has not been easy. It's been bumpy. Celebrate what you have done, and feel good about this accomplishment.

Six weeks ago, you might have doubted you could make it through the first day. But today you have overcome the struggle of 40 days! This is a monumental event. This time has been the preview—not the main event! It has prepared you for what you are about to do. To continue to succeed, you must remember everything you've been taught. You can't allow it to be something you "did." It must be something you "live!"

Transformation is about lifestyle and sustaining habits that align with your New You visions, dreams and aspirations. You are like a runner. At the starting line, he takes off to run his race. He runs. He exerts himself lap after lap. He does all he can to finish victoriously. And, he crosses the finish line with great joy and exhilaration. The strange truth about the runner is that the starting line becomes the finish line! The race begins and ends at the same place!

Today, although you are celebrating what you have done and your "finish," when you think about it, you are now back at the starting line! Don't view this as the end of the process but rather as the start of another season in your life. Keep pressing forward! Shalom

TAKE AWAY

Don't allow these 40 days to be something you "did." Let them be something you continue to "live!" Keep pressing forward!

CHALLENGE

Think back through the last 40 days. What are some of the most powerful things you've learned about yourself and this process? What truths will be most helpful to you in continuing to live out this new lifestyle?

_____

_____   **THOUGHTS,**
                                                    PRAYERS, &
_____   **REFLECTIONS**

_____

_____

_____

_____

_____

_____

_____

_____

_____

_____

_____